A Bill Of Rights
For
Periodic Paralysis Patients

From

The Periodic Paralysis Network A.S.E.A. Series

Awareness ~ Support ~ Education ~ Advocacy

Volume One

Susan Q. Knittle-Hunter
&
Calvin Hunter

A Bill Of Rights For Periodic Paralysis Patients
From
The Periodic Paralysis Network A.S.E.A. Series
Volume One
By
Susan Q. Knittle-Hunter
&
Calvin Hunter

Periodic Paralysis Network, Inc.
Sequim, Washington U.S.A.

Copyright © 2015
Library of Congress Cataloging-in-Publication Data:
A Bill Of Rights For Periodic Paralysis Patients
From
The Periodic Paralysis Network A.S.E.A. Series
Volume One
By
Susan Q. Knittle-Hunter
&
Calvin Hunter

First Edition
ISBN-13: 978-1517196233
ISBN-10: 151719623X
1. Andersen-Tawil Syndrome 2. Periodic Paralysis 3. Hypokalemia
4. Hyperkalemia 5. Normokalemia 6. Hypokalemic Periodic Paralysis
7. Hyperkalemic Periodic Paralysis
Printed in the United States of America.
2015

Notice-Disclaimer
The ideas in this book are based on the authors' personal experiences with Periodic Paralysis, and as such are intended to provide only educational information on the covered subject to the reader. This book should not be used as a medical manual nor should this book be used as a diagnostic tool for Periodic Paralysis. The reader should consult a qualified health care professional or physician with expertise in Periodic Paralysis.

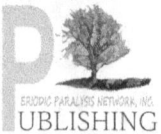

Periodic Paralysis Network, Inc. Publishing
Sequim, Washington U.S.A.
2015

This booklet is dedicated to the members of the 'Periodic Paralysis Network Support, Education and Advocacy Group'…May you receive the treatment and respect you deserve from the medical professionals involved in your care.

*"As to diseases, make a habit of two things —
to help, or at least, to do no harm."*

Hippocrates
Father of Medicine

Table of Contents

About A.S.E.A.   vi
Preface   viii
Acknowledgements   ix
Introduction   x
What is a Bill of Rights?   13
The General Rights   29
The Diagnosis of Periodic Paralysis   41
Treatment in the Laboratory   55
Treatment by Doctors   63
Treatment in the ER and Hospital   75
Research and Awareness   99
Insurance   105
Conclusion   109
Periodic Paralysis Forum   110
About the Authors   111

**About
The Periodic Paralysis Network
A.S.E.A. Series:**

Awareness ~ Support ~ Education ~ Advocacy

Volume One

A Bill Of Rights For Periodic Paralysis Patients is the first volume in a series of booklets or handbooks being created, written and published by the Periodic Paralysis Network, Inc. (PPN). This series, called *The Periodic Paralysis Network A.S.E.A. Series*, is designed to bring awareness of Periodic Paralysis to the world; to provide support to individuals with all forms of Periodic Paralysis and their family members; to educate individuals about all aspects of Periodic Paralysis to include medical professionals and to provide advocacy for those with the condition and their family members and caregivers. The PPN was created and exists to provide **A**wareness, **S**upport, **E**ducation and **A**dvocacy to and for all individuals with Periodic Paralysis, their family members and caregivers as well as all medical professionals, thus the acronym A.S.E.A.

We begin this series with a bill of rights for patients with Periodic Paralysis.

Also by Susan Q. Knittle-Hunter & Calvin Hunter

living with Periodic Paralysis: The Mystery Unraveled

*The Periodic Paralysis Guide And Workbook:
Be All You Can Be Naturally*

Also by Susan Q. Knittle-Hunter

Sotos Syndrome: A Tribute To Sandy

Also by Calvin Hunter

Moments In Time: At Home In The Woods

Preface

The Preface of a book gives the reader information about how the book came to be, where the idea originated. In the case of this booklet, the members of the 'Periodic Paralysis Network Support, Education and Advocacy Group' inspired *A Bill of Rights For Periodic Paralysis Patients.* The members, now over 425 worldwide, share daily their heart-breaking and frustrating experiences. They relate frightening symptoms, years of painful and costly testing, a lack of being believed, abuse by doctors, denial of diagnoses and denial of proper treatment. These courageous and very ill people are under-recognized, under-diagnosed, mis-diagnosed, mis-under-stood and mistreated by the medical professionals with whom they must deal and depend upon for their care. Their general rights; diagnostic rights; the right to proper treatment in the laboratory, by doctors and in the ER; the right to research and awareness and issues related to insurance rights have been and are being violated in many cases. This needs to stop.

For these reasons a bill of rights for individuals with Periodic Paralysis has been created, by the PPN. The information used to outline, describe and explain these concepts and rights are referenced and can be found at the Periodic Paralysis Network, Inc. Website, Blog Articles, Discussion Groups and Books.

Acknowledgements

We would like to thank the members of our Periodic Paralysis Network Support, Education and Advocacy Group. Each one of them has inspired us in more ways than they could possibly know. We created our forum to help others who suffer daily from the cruel and unusual effects of the many forms and mutations of Periodic Paralysis. We had hoped to give support to others that we did not receive as we searched for help. We hoped to provide easy to understand, up-to-date and accurate information in one place about all aspects of Periodic Paralysis, which we were unable to find. Lastly, we hoped to be advocates for correct, honest, appropriate and safe treatment, which we were unable to locate and experience. After five years, we are so happy that our forum has grown and we now are able to provide these things for our worldwide members.

What we did not expect or anticipate was the way in which the members of our group have become our friends and return to us much more than we give and have given them. We receive support and encouragement on bad days, we learn something new every day from them as they share their information and stories and they are advocates for us in all ways.

Thank you so much for your strength, words of encouragement, support and love. We could not do it all without each of you.

Introduction

As discussed in the Preface and for the reasons listed, there was and is a great need for a bill of rights for all individuals who have a form of the metabolic disorder known as Periodic Paralysis. The Periodic Paralysis Network, inspired by the members of the 'Periodic Paralysis Network Support, Education and Advocacy Group' has now created *A Bill of Rights For Periodic Paralysis Patients*. This booklet, the first in the PPN A.S.E.A. Series, begins with an explanation of what a 'bill of rights' is and why they are written or created.

Next, '*A Bill of Rights For Periodic Paralysis Patients*' is outlined in seven sections, covering general rights, diagnosis, treatment in labs, treatment by doctors and treatment in the emergency room and the areas of research, awareness and insurance. In those, each concept is described and explained based on the true and actual history, experiences and needs of individuals with Periodic Paralysis.

Hopefully, this information will bring about awareness of these issues and educate everyone who has the occasion to read this booklet as well as the medical professionals with whom individuals with Periodic Paralysis must depend upon to insure correct and proper care. By pointing out the wrongs, it is greatly desired that these wrongs can be made right and corrected.

More information and referencing can be found at the Periodic Paralysis Network Inc Website, Blog Articles, discussion groups and books; *Living With Periodic Paralysis: The Mystery Unraveled* and *The Periodic Paralysis Guide And Workbook: Be The Best You Can Be Naturally*.

What is a Bill of Rights?

A Bill of Rights

A 'bill of rights' may also be called a 'charter of rights' or a 'declaration of rights.' It is a list of ethical, social or legal principles of entitlements or freedoms or what could be referred to as that which is "owed" to an individual. Bills of rights exist from lists of basic human rights worldwide to lists of a country's or a state's citizen's rights. A declaration of rights has been created for all patient's in the United States health system and all hospitals have a bill of rights for their patients. Specifically, targeted groups such as stroke victims, individuals with multiple sclerosis and cancer patients have bills of rights. Until now, however, no bill of rights has been created for individuals with Periodic Paralysis. This is a group of very ill people who are under-recognized; under-diagnosed, mis-diagnosed, misunderstood and mistreated by the medical professionals with whom they must deal and depend upon for their care. It is time for a Periodic Paralysis Patient's Bill of Rights.

First it must be understood that there exists basic medical ethics; called a 'code of ethics,' which is a set of moral principles. Physicians around the world follow these guidelines found in the Hippocratic oath. They take this sworn pledge before they begin to practice medicine. The following are the principles typically included:

~A doctor must have the best interest of the patient
~A doctor's treatment must be based on equality and fairness
~A doctor must "do no harm"
~A doctor's treatment may be accepted or refused by the patient
~A doctor must treat patients with dignity
~A doctor must be honest and truthful

National Patient's Bills of Rights

In 1998 the US Advisory Commission on Consumer Protection and Quality in the Health Care Industry created and adopted what is known as the Patient's Bill of Rights, a summary of principles. There are three major goals:

~To assist patients to feel more confidence in the United States health care system

~To stress a strong association and connection between health care providers and their patients

~To stress the importance for patients to stay healthy

Individuals are entitled to eight major components in the National Patient's Bills of Rights related to insurance plans and hospitals (including emergency care):

A patient is entitled to:

~Accurate and easy-to-understand information about one's health plan, medical professionals and facilities for health care

~Choice of the best health care provider for a particular medical condition

~Access to services for emergencies

~Being a member of the team for making all individual health care choices

~Respect and considerate treatment, with a lack of discrimination, from all healthcare workers

~Privacy and confidentiality and the right to copy and read all medical records and to change anything that is incorrect or not relevant and to add to records which are not complete

~Complain and make appeals about any medical care provider, regarding waiting time, actions or non-actions and adequacy of services or facilities

The above goals and components have been adopted and are used by Medicare, Medicaid, hospitals, insurance companies, long-term medical facilities and more. They are the basis for targeted medical groups bills of rights also.

Using these principles of basic entitlement combined with the needs of individuals with Periodic Paralysis, the following bill of rights has been created.

Note:
The reader will find some redundancy or repetition of some issues. This is because there is an overlap of several issues across each of the categories.

A Bill of Rights
for
Periodic Paralysis Patients

Outlined

A Bill of Rights for Periodic Paralysis Patients

The General Rights

The right to be the team leader of one's own medical care, needs and decisions ~

The right to be treated with respect and dignity by all medical professionals~

The right for the symptoms of muscle weakness and/or paralysis and any other pertinent issues to be taken seriously~

The right to be treated as anyone else is treated who has a chronic, disabling medical condition~

The right for medical professionals to understand that Periodic Paralysis is a mineral metabolic disorder (channelopathy), not a neurological or muscle disease and should not be treated as such~

The right for all medical professionals to understand that Periodic Paralysis is like no other medical condition and needs to be treated like no other medical condition~

The right for all medical professionals to understand that Periodic Paralysis exists in several forms and may present with low potassium, high potassium or potassium within normal levels~

The right for all medical professionals to be educated about all aspects of Periodic Paralysis including all forms, the symptoms for each and the treatment for each~

The right for Social Security Disability to recognize Periodic Paralysis as a chronic, disabling condition~

Diagnosis of Periodic Paralysis

The right to a timely diagnosis~

The right to a clinical diagnosis based on symptoms as in every other disease and medical condition~

The right for Whole Genome DNA Testing to be paid for by insurance~

The right for doctors to understand that only about 50% of Periodic Paralysis genetic mutations have been discovered, so a negative DNA test result does rule out Periodic Paralysis~

The right for any type of doctor to diagnose Periodic Paralysis~

The right to refuse provocative testing for diagnosing Periodic Paralysis~

The right for a doctor to believe a diagnosis of Periodic Paralysis~

The right to maintain a diagnosis for Periodic Paralysis once it has been given, no doctor has a right to change or dismiss a diagnosis~

The right for doctors to understand that other medical conditions may co-exist with Periodic Paralysis~

The right for doctors to understand that potassium may not shift out of normal ranges during paralytic episodes or other symptoms~

The right to not be diagnosed with a mental or somatic disorder because a doctor does not understand or believe in Periodic Paralysis~

The right to not be diagnosed with Periodic Paralysis because it is considered "too rare"~

Treatment in The Laboratory

The right to be treated with respect and dignity by lab technicians~

The right to have blood drawn with no tourniquets~

The right to have blood drawn as quickly as possible, even if it means going out to the car to draw the blood or to a patient's home~

The right to know the potassium level as quickly as possible using an ISTAT or potassium reader~

The right for staff to understand that normal potassium levels do not rule out Periodic Paralysis~

Treatment by Doctors and Medical Professionals

The right to be treated with respect and dignity by doctors and all medical professionals~

The right for the symptoms of muscle weakness and/or paralysis and other pertinent issues to be taken seriously by the doctors~

The right for the symptoms of muscle weakness and/or paralysis and other pertinent issues to be thoroughly assessed and treated promptly as needed~

The right to dismiss a doctor for inappropriate care, lack of knowledge of Periodic Paralysis and poor attitude~

The right to refuse any and all drugs prescribed by a doctor; to include IV's and anesthesia~

The right for clear, concise and truthful medical notes and records to be written by the doctors and other medical professionals~

The right to read and receive copies of all medical records and the right to challenge, add to and to change their content if not accurate~

The right to complain and make appeals about any doctor or medical care provider, regarding waiting time, actions or non-actions and adequacy of services~

The right to be referred to a doctor who understands Periodic Paralysis~

Treatment in the ER and Hospital

The right to be treated with respect and dignity by doctors and medical professionals~

The right to be seen quickly~

The right to be comfortable and safe~

The right to be accompanied and observed constantly by medical staff when in a paralytic episode~

The right for the doctors and medical professionals to

listen to the patient (if possible), family members or caregivers on instruction for care~

The right for the doctors and medical professionals to read information provided by the patient, family members or caregivers on how to care for the patient~

The right for all doctors and medical professionals to follow the specific instructions provided, to include proper positioning, no IV's, no drugs and more, as necessary~

The right to have blood drawn with no tourniquets for potassium levels which may indicate potassium levels that may be low, high or within normal ranges~

The right to have blood drawn as quickly as possible preferably using a potassium reader or ISTAT for instant results which may indicate potassium levels that may be low, high or within normal ranges~

The right for the symptoms of muscle weakness and/or paralysis, and other pertinent issues to be thoroughly assessed~

The right for the symptoms of muscle weakness and/or paralysis and others as pertinent, to be taken seriously by the doctors and medical care professionals~

The right to be observed for choking, heart arrhythmia, fluctuations in blood pressure, and heart rate, breathing issues, low oxygen levels and others as pertinent~

The right to not be harmed during paralysis by doctors or other medical professionals attempting to prove "faking" by pinching, scratching, burning or sticking with pins or needles~

The right to be treated for choking, heart arrhythmia, fluctuations in blood pressure, and heart rate, breathing issues, low oxygen levels as pertinent~

The right to refuse IV's, drugs, medications and anesthesia, which may be harmful or deadly~

The right to refuse provocative testing for the reason of diagnosing Periodic Paralysis~

The right to call in a hospitalist, or other specialists who may know about Periodic Paralysis as needed~

The right to call in a social worker or patient advocate as needed~

The right to dismiss a doctor or other medical professional for inappropriate care, lack of knowledge of Periodic Paralysis and poor attitude~

The right for clear, concise and truthful medical notes and records to be written by the doctors and other medical professionals~

The right to read and receive copies of all medical records and the right to challenge, add to and to change their content if not accurate~

The right to complain and make appeals about any doctor or medical care provider, regarding waiting time, actions or non-actions and adequacy of service~

Research and Awareness

The right to increase the awareness of Periodic Paralysis among populations, doctors and governments~

The right to "put a face" to Periodic Paralysis as in other known diseases and medical conditions~

The right for all medical professionals to be educated about all aspects of Periodic Paralysis including all forms, the symptoms for each and the appropriate treatment for each~

The right to funding for research of all aspects of Periodic Paralysis including but not limited to diagnosis and treatment~

Insurance

The right for all forms of Periodic Paralysis to be recognized as disabling conditions by insurance companies~

The right for potassium readers to be deemed as medical devices and paid for by insurance companies~

The right to have ISTAT devices for monitoring vitals for all Periodic Paralysis patients and to have them paid for by insurance companies~

The right for the special natural and organic diet and supplementation that must be followed by patients with Periodic Paralysis to be paid for in part by insurance companies~

A Bill of Rights
for
Periodic Paralysis Patients

Each concept is described and explained based on the true and actual history, experiences and needs of individuals with Periodic Paralysis.

The General Rights

The General Rights

~The right to be the team leader of one's own medical care, needs and decisions~

Periodic Paralysis (PP) is a mineral metabolic disorder that is commonly diagnosed after everything else has been ruled out so it takes an average of twenty years to obtain a diagnosis. This is usually after innumerable medical tests and examinations, scores of visits to doctors and medical professionals, countless wrong diagnoses and dozens of improper medications and treatment. After decades of this pattern, an individual with any form of Periodic Paralysis may very well know more about Periodic Paralysis and his or her own body than the doctors and medical professionals they must see for diagnosis and treatment.

Therefore, the patient needs to be in control of the medical team and direct all of the players who may consist of a primary care physician (PCP), neurologists, endocrinologists, nephrologists, allergists internists, cardiologists, rheumatologists, dentists urologists, geneticists, psychiatrists, ophthalmologists, physical therapists, counselors, social workers, nurses, radiologists, lab technicians, EMT's, paramedics, family members, caregivers and more. The individual must express his or her needs and desires based on symptoms, triggers, changes, complications from treatments and side effects from drugs and medications. He or she then has the right to make medical decisions that are in his or her best interest based on research, education, information, test results, past experience and personal preference.

An individual with Periodic Paralysis must coordinate and lead his or her own medical team for diagnosis, treatment and care.

~The right to be treated with respect and dignity by all medical professionals~

The episodes of paralysis or muscle weakness can look "fake" to medical professionals and others. Years of medical testing may reveal no diagnosis. Genetic testing, which is limited and narrow may also be negative for Periodic Paralysis. Due to this, many patients report verbal and mental abuse from their doctors, nurses, technicians and other medical professionals who do not understand the metabolic condition.

Though unbelievable, individuals with Periodic Paralysis, before receiving a diagnosis and some even after, have been lied to; lied about in records; called names; yelled at; watched doctors throw things in anger; hurt while in paralysis when a doctor is trying to prove they are "faking" by scratching, pinching or sticking with pins; refused meds they need; given drugs they do not need; left alone like a naughty child while in paralysis to be punished for bad behavior; scoffed at; laughed at; made to cry; been belittled; told they are "too old" to have the condition and much more. This should never have happened and must not happen in the future.

All medical professionals must treat every patient with Periodic Paralysis, or possible Periodic Paralysis, with respect and dignity just like every other patient with any "more known" medical conditions.

~The right for the symptoms of muscle weakness and/or paralysis and any other pertinent issues to be taken seriously~

Medical records indicating decades of odd and severe symptoms, which may appear "fake", medical tests that are always negative, visits to every type of doctor that exists, medications with uncommon side effects, progressive muscle weakness and more are presented to a patient's present doctors or to new doctors who do not know about or understand Periodic Paralysis. These physicians almost immediately begin to view the patient as having mental issues and doubt that a medical issue exists. Words begin to appear in the medical notes with terms like "somatic" or "conversion disorder."

The patient is given drugs for anxiety, depression or psychosis, which causes new symptoms, more paralysis and harmful side effects including the possibility of death. He or she is then dismissed and the symptoms disregarded. He or she is not taken seriously. The patient becomes more ill, and family and friends begin to also dismiss the claims of illness. The patient is expected to continue on with life duties and responsibilities though he or she progressively gets worse. This is wrong and every patient with Periodic Paralysis or the possibility of Periodic Paralysis needs to be taken seriously.

~The right to be treated as anyone else is treated who has a chronic, disabling medical condition~

Periodic Paralysis is a very rare, but real, chronic and serious medical condition known as an ion channelopathy or a mineral metabolic disorder. In most cases it causes progressive and permanent muscle weakness. If treated incorrectly individuals may be harmed or die. There are several forms and each can be very disabling sometimes requiring the use of canes, walkers or wheelchairs. It is as real as multiple sclerosis, diabetes, muscular dystrophy, cancer and Parkinson's disease. It is just not as well known; in fact it is not known or understood by most medical professionals. Every patient with Periodic Paralysis or who is suspected of having Periodic Paralysis has the right to be diagnosed and treated just like anyone else with a chronic and disabling medical condition.

~The right for medical professionals to understand that Periodic Paralysis is a mineral metabolic disorder (channelopathy), not a neurological or muscle disease and should not be treated as such~

As stated previously, most medical professionals do not know about or understand much about Periodic Paralysis. Because the symptoms look like a neurological condition, patients are sent to neurologists for testing and diagnosis. The doctors will prescribe drugs to treat symptoms that look neurological and new symptoms and harmful side effects will develop due to the nature of a channelopathy. Test after test will be performed, which result in normal findings. Once all testing is complete and all neurological conditions are ruled out, a diagnosis of Periodic Paralysis should be given. Another problem is that the Muscular Dystrophy Association (MDA) lists it as one of their diseases because it affects muscles, but it is not a form of muscular dystrophy. Periodic Paralysis is a mineral metabolic disorder also known as a channelopathy.

An ion channelopathy is a dysfunction of an ion channel, a microscopic tunnel in the cells of muscles called muscle fibers. Particles of potassium, sodium, chloride or calcium, which are electrically charged, known as ions, flow in and out of the cells. They regulate the contraction and relaxation of the muscle. A problem with the flow can cause paralysis.

Periodic Paralysis is not a neurological condition nor is it a form of muscular dystrophy. Treating it as either may be harmful or deadly to the patient.

~The right for all medical professionals to understand that Periodic Paralysis is like no other medical condition and needs to be treated like no other medical condition~

Because Periodic Paralysis is a channelopathy or what is also called a mineral metabolic disorder, the basics and problems with this condition happen on a cellular level. Potassium shifts in error either 'in,' 'into' or 'out of' the muscles causing many possible symptoms and of course periods of temporary paralysis or muscle weakness. The individual rarely loses consciousness and can hear everything going on around him or her. The paralysis may be full body or partial paralysis, affecting only one limb or more than one part of the body. The episodes may last minutes, hours or possibly days.

It is not a muscle disease nor a neurological disease and cannot be treated with drugs used for those conditions. In fact most drugs, IVs and anesthesia are harmful and can cause serious symptoms and trigger the paralytic episodes. During these attacks besides paralysis, there may be serious heart arrhythmia, fluctuating heart rate and blood pressure, choking, breathing issues and low oxygen levels. A patient may stop breathing or go into coronary or respiratory arrest or both and therefore, the patient must never be left alone during an episode and all vitals must be constantly monitored.

Drugs, food, salt, sugar, gluten, stress, sleep, exercise and many more things can trigger the symptoms. So treatment for Periodic Paralysis usually centers on natural methods to include discovering and avoiding the triggers and following a balanced diet. Doctors need to understand that Periodic Paralysis is not like any other medical condition and must be treated differently.

~The right for all medical professionals to understand that Periodic Paralysis exists in several forms and may present with low potassium, high potassium or potassium within normal levels~

The several forms or types of Periodic Paralysis follow:

Hypokalemic Periodic Paralysis (HypoPP):
Paralysis results from potassium moving from the blood into muscle cells in an abnormal way. It is associated with low levels of potassium in the blood (hypokalemia) during paralytic episodes.

Hyperkalemic Periodic Paralysis (HyperPP):
Paralysis results from problems with the way the body controls sodium and potassium levels in cells. It is associated with high levels of potassium in the blood (hyperkalemia) during paralytic episodes.

Andersen-Tawil Syndrome (ATS):
Paralysis results when the channel does not open properly, potassium cannot leave the cell. This disrupts the flow of potassium ions in skeletal and cardiac muscle. During paralytic episodes, ATS can be associated with low potassium, high potassium or shifts within the normal (normokalemia) ranges of potassium. An arrhythmia, long Qt interval heartbeat, is associated with ATS as well as certain characteristics, such as webbed or partially webbed toes, crooked little fingers and dental anomalies.

Normokalemic Periodic Paralysis (NormoPP):
Paralysis results when potassium shifts within in normal ranges. This can happen in any form of Periodic Paralysis; Hypokalemic Periodic Paralysis,

Hyperkalemic Periodic Paralysis, Normokalemic Periodic Paralysis and Andersen-Tawil Syndrome.The paralysis may result from the shifting itself, rather than low or high potassium or it may occur due to the shifting of the potassium, which can happen very quickly and is undetectable in lab testing.

Paramyotonia Congenita (PMC):

The skeletal muscles can become stiff, tight, tense or contracted and weak due when the sodium channels close much too slowly and the sodium, potassium, chloride and water continue to flow into the muscles. It is actually considered to be a form of Hyperkalemic Periodic Paralysis, however, the symptoms can appear from shifting of potassium into low or high ranges or even if potassium shifts within normal levels.

Thyrotoxic Periodic Paralysis (TPP):

Intermittent paralysis results from low potassium due to an overactive thyroid or hyperthyroidism. It can occur spontaneously or can result from a genetic mutation. Unlike the other forms of Periodic Paralysis, TPP can be treated and cured by removing or treating the thyroid.

~

~The right for all medical professionals to be educated about all aspects of Periodic Paralysis including all forms, the symptoms for each and the treatment for each~

It takes nearly a decade of graduate school to become a doctor. During those years of training, Periodic Paralysis is mentioned in one or two paragraphs and in those paragraphs it is described as so rare that a doctor will never see a patient with it in his or her lifetime or years of practice. This is a serious disservice to those of us who have the condition.

As it turns out Periodic Paralysis is not all that "rare," but rather it is under-recognized and under-diagnosed and mis-diagnosed. As stated before it takes an average of twenty years for an individual to receive a diagnosis. Many die before they ever receive a diagnosis. This is unconscionable and unnecessary. This would not be the case if all medical professionals understood Periodic Paralysis and knew how to recognize this condition.

More education and training is needed for students in medical school and for all other medical professionals including nurses, EMT's, paramedics, social workers, teachers, lab technicians and more. Periodic Paralysis needs to be as commonly understood as other medical conditions such as multiple sclerosis, muscular dystrophy, fibromyalgia, heart disease, diabetes, and Lou Gehrig's disease.

~The right for Social Security Disability to recognize Periodic Paralysis as a chronic, disabling condition~

The majority of individuals who have Periodic Paralysis develop permanent muscle weakness, autoimmune conditions or dysfunction and/or even mitochondrial conditions or dysfunction before they ever get a confirmed diagnosis. Although Periodic Paralysis is on the list of medical diseases and conditions generally accepted as disabling enough for which to receive disabilities services, when applying for Social Security Disability, an individual will more than likely be granted disability or be deemed disabled based on a misdiagnosis, an autoimmune condition or a mitochondrial condition most likely caused from the untreated or mistreated Periodic Paralysis, rather than the actual diagnosis.

Periodic Paralysis needs to be recognized and diagnosed in a much more timely manner so that it can be the actual condition for which one is granted Social Security Disability. This is to insure proper treatment and follow-up. The doctors who are hired to evaluate the patients seeking Social Security Disability must know about and understand Periodic Paralysis in order to provide a correct diagnosis. It needs to be recognized for the chronic and disabling condition that it is.

The Diagnosis of Periodic Paralysis

The Diagnosis of Periodic Paralysis

~The right to a timely diagnosis~

Studies indicate that it takes an average of twenty years and is certainly very costly for someone with Periodic Paralysis to get a diagnosis. This is ludicrous and unconscionable. During those years an individual's symptoms worsen. He or she develops exercise intolerance, permanent muscle weakness, heart issues and breathing issues and is harmed from unnecessary drugs and medications. Some may even die needlessly.

This creates the destruction of the quality of an individual's life, leading to a possible loss of family, friends, job, finances, home, self-esteem and much more. Without a diagnosis, the ability to get disability and proper care diminishes.

Those twenty years or more consist of seeing doctor after doctor, specialist after specialist; taking test after test, because it is a condition in which a diagnosis is obtained by exclusion, it is diagnosed after everything else is ruled out. Since very few medical conditions actually cause a person to have intermittent paralysis and/or muscle weakness, after those few conditions are ruled out, it should not take much time to then diagnoses Periodic Paralysis.

Some people are still waiting over fifty or sixty years for a diagnosis. No one should have to wait a lifetime for a diagnosis and proper treatment.

Periodic Paralysis needs to be diagnosed clinically, based on symptoms, in a timely manner for the proper care and treatment of the condition and for the well being mentally, psychologically and physically of the patient.

~The right to a clinical diagnosis based on symptoms as in every other disease and medical condition~

Most medical conditions and diseases are well known, easily recognized and diagnosed based on their symptoms and characteristics in a timely manner. This is usually done very routinely through testing, which may include but not limited to X-rays, MRI's, blood tests, urine tests, biopsies, and EKG's. Some conditions are diagnosed through genetic testing and the mutations are very well known, easily found and quite obvious.

For many reasons, not well understood, Periodic Paralysis has been made very difficult to diagnose and takes an average of twenty years. In the beginning it was believed that without positive genetic test results, an individual did not have the condition. As discussed earlier, it is now known that this is not correct. One-half of individuals with Periodic Paralysis have a form for which no mutation has been discovered as yet. Unfortunately, it is common today for doctors to still believe that 'no genetic code' equals 'no' diagnosis. They refuse to diagnose based on the obvious symptoms, after all else has been ruled out.

The other issue of denying a diagnosis is based on out-dated information. That is, if the potassium does not shift into a low or high range than PP does not exist. This is totally wrong. The potassium does not have to shift out of normal range for muscle weakness or paralysis to occur.

Obtaining a clinical diagnosis, based on obvious symptoms, is essential. Once it is on paper, individuals are at least believed for emergency care issues, hospitalizations, possible medications, school issues for children, insurance, validation, vindication, disability and much more.

~The right for Whole Genome DNA Testing to be paid for by insurance~

As recently as a year ago, genetic testing for Periodic Paralysis was performed in Germany for free, but the cost to get it there was not cheap. Patients waited for a year to several years for the results. That testing, however, was narrow and biased because not every form was sequenced. Due to the fact that only fifty percent of those with PP have a mutation that has been discovered, the results were very limited and misleading. Many very ill individuals were lead to believe that they did not have the condition. The testing was discontinued not long ago.

The only testing now available is through private labs at great cost. Those tests are also very limited, especially when ordered by a doctor with little or misinformed knowledge about the many mutations and types of Periodic Paralysis. They tend to order testing for one or two particular mutations.

The best way to obtain a genetic diagnosis presently, with the understanding that new or undiscovered genetic mutations may not be found or recognized, is to have Whole Genome DNA Sequencing done. The problem with this is the cost. Most insurance companies will not pay for it.

Individuals with the symptoms of Periodic Paralysis deserve the right to Whole Genome Testing, the right for it to be ordered by their physicians and the right for it to be paid for by their insurance companies.

~The right for doctors to understand that only about 50% of Periodic Paralysis genetic mutations have been discovered, so a negative DNA test result does rule out Periodic Paralysis~

Because only about one half of the genetic mutations for the forms of Periodic Paralysis are actually known and because most testing ordered by doctors is very narrow and limited, usually testing for one or two particular forms or mutations and because even Whole Genetic Testing may miss or not uncover the genetic mutation responsible for an individual's Periodic Paralysis symptoms, doctors need to understand that not everyone who has Periodic Paralysis will be able to obtain a diagnosis through genetic testing. Doctors, who do not understand this, have and do, assume that negative results clearly indicate that an individual does not have a form of Periodic Paralysis.

At this point diagnosing the condition needs to be done clinically, that is, based on symptoms and characteristics. Unfortunately, most doctors do not know about Periodic Paralysis and they do not recognize the symptoms and so it takes decades because all other conditions must be ruled out unless the signs of low potassium or high potassium are present, and even then it is often dismissed as the possible cause for paralysis or weakness.

Doctors need to be educated about all aspects of Periodic Paralysis so that it is easily recognized, to include that not everyone will have a known genetic mutation revealed during testing and research needs to continue to find the forms yet to be discovered.

~The right for any type of doctor to diagnose Periodic Paralysis~

Due to the fact that the symptoms of Periodic Paralysis look neurological in nature, patients with this condition are traditionally referred to neurologists for testing, treatment and diagnosis. Once all testing has been completed, and all other conditions have been ruled out, then a diagnosis of Periodic Paralysis should be given. However, that is not what happens. Neurologists at this point begin to believe the symptoms may be 'somatic' or 'not real' and a diagnosis of 'conversion disorder' is then placed on the patient.

This is unfortunate indeed, because Periodic Paralysis is not a neurological disorder, but rather a mineral metabolic disorder. It is unlike any other medical condition and needs to be treated differently than any other condition. Due to this fact, any type of doctor can diagnose it. If a doctor knows about Periodic Paralysis and recognizes it and after a neurologist or other doctors has ruled everything else out, he or she can and SHOULD diagnose it.

Using natural methods and common sense is the best treatment and management for the symptoms. Drugs, IV's and anesthesia must be avoided for nearly all forms. With this knowledge, any type of doctor should be able to help or direct his or her patient to manage the symptoms and paralytic episodes.

~The right to refuse provocative testing for diagnosing Periodic Paralysis ~

It was discovered some time back that due to the nature of a mineral metabolic disorder, there were things that could trigger the symptoms of muscle weakness and paralysis. These triggers, depending on the particular form of Periodic Paralysis, include but are not limited to, most drugs, IV's (glucose and saline), anesthesia, salt, sugar, potassium, gluten, food fillers and dyes, sleep, exercise, cold, heat and stress.

Doctors, not understanding the serious implications of being in a paralytic episode including dangerous heart arrhythmia (even possibly long QT heart beats), dangerous heart rate and blood pressure fluctuations, low oxygen levels, choking, breathing cessation, cardiac and respiratory arrest and possible death; decided that in order to prove or disprove the existence of the condition, could "provoke" the symptoms and paralysis by putting a patient on an IV of glucose and then when the symptoms begin, quickly give them potassium to stop it.

Because some forms of Periodic Paralysis are just the opposite or react in different ways, some of these patients died. Provoking an attack of paralysis is NEVER to be done. It is far too risky and can end in death.

Any and every patient with Periodic Paralysis has the right to refuse the provocation of his or her symptoms by a doctor or other medical care professional.

~The right for a doctor to believe a diagnosis of Periodic Paralysis~

Once an individual has been given a diagnosis for Periodic Paralysis he or she has the right for that diagnosis to be believed by the other physicians or medical professionals he or she may need to see. No doctor has the right to question it or scoff at it because they do not understand it. If a doctor does not believe it or understand Periodic Paralysis or does not believe the patient has it, he or she needs to remove himself or herself from the situation or the patient has the right to dismiss him or her as the acting physician.

A patient needs to be safe and a doctor, who does not or will not believe or understand the diagnosis, may harm the patient with improper treatment.

~The right to maintain a diagnosis for Periodic Paralysis once it has been given, no doctor has a right to change or dismiss a diagnosis~

As stated earlier, once an individual has been given a diagnosis for Periodic Paralysis he or she has the right for that diagnosis to be believed by the other physicians or medical professionals he or she may need to see.

Many individuals with Periodic Paralysis have been diagnosed clinically, based on the characteristics, symptoms and periods of paralysis or muscle weakness. At this point they wish to see 'specialists' with the hope of improving the quality of their lives. After much difficulty in securing appointments, borrowing money to travel across the country and all the while in and out of paralysis, 'specialists' will see these individuals. Many of them, due to age, co-existing conditions and/or atypical symptoms, will be humiliated and have their diagnoses overturned. Many of them later get diagnosed through genetic testing. In some cases, thank goodness, the referring and/or diagnosing physicians throw the reports from the 'specialists' into the trash. But not all doctors realize the terrible mistake that has been made and follow the lead of the 'specialists.' This is very detrimental to the patient.

Once an individual has received a diagnosis for Periodic Paralysis, it needs to stand because as stated previously, obtaining a clinical diagnosis, based on our obvious symptoms, is essential. Once it is on paper, individuals are at least believed for emergency care issues, hospitalizations, possible medications, school issues for children, insurance, validation, vindication, disability and much more.

~The right for doctors to understand that other medical conditions may co-exist with Periodic Paralysis~

Research indicates that mineral metabolic disorders, like Periodic Paralysis, can create mitochondrial dysfunction or conditions. Mitochondrial dysfunction can then create autoimmune dysfunction or disorders. Therefore, any individual with a form of Periodic Paralysis has a chance of also developing both mitochondrial issues and autoimmune issues, especially the older they become and the longer they are without proper treatment. It is further known that genetic mutations on a specific chromosome may cause issues or mutations on other areas of that chromosome. Many genetic mutations of Periodic Paralysis are located on chromosome 17. It is not uncommon for other genetic conditions found on that chromosome to co-exist with Periodic Paralysis. Furthermore, out-dated and erroneous information exists, which states that patients with Periodic Paralysis do not experience pain.

Some doctors and 'specialists' refuse to diagnose an individual if they have coexisting conditions or if they experience pain. These doctors need to be educated and brought up-to-date with the latest information about Periodic Paralysis. Anyone can have more than one rare condition and pain can and does exist in patients with Periodic Paralysis. A diagnosis should not be withheld, based on these issues.

With each wrong diagnosis and wrong medication individuals get sicker, more damage is done to the organs and permanent muscle weakness sets in. We risk death each time we go into paralysis. This is inexcusable.

~The right for doctors to understand that potassium may not shift out of normal ranges during paralytic episodes or other symptoms~

It is erroneous to believe that an individual does not have Periodic Paralysis because their potassium level does not drop or rise during an episode of muscle weakness or paralysis. As described previously there are several forms of the condition and each creates the symptoms in a different manner. Some patients may have low potassium levels; some high potassium levels and some may have normal levels of potassium during an episode. There are several reasons for this.

The potassium may shift very quickly and may not be caught on a lab test, after the fact. Also, there are forms, which do not shift at all out of the normal range, they are known as 'Normokalemic Periodic Paralysis' and recent studies indicate that in the varying forms of Periodic Paralysis the main problem is that the normal pores do not work correctly in the muscle cells. Potassium levels can affect this but it is not necessary for a change in the potassium level in the blood to create muscle weakness or paralysis.

So, because doctors do not understand these concepts, and again due to out-dated and erroneous information, many patients are either not diagnosed due to normal potassium levels accompanying symptoms or they are refused treatment in an ER or the patient is believed to be 'faking' or lying. This puts a person with Periodic Paralysis at risk for harm from improper treatment or a lack of proper treatment. This is a serious issue and needs to be changed. It is obvious that many doctors need to be trained appropriately regarding all aspects of Periodic Paralysis, especially the issue of normal levels of potassium during an episode of periodic paralysis.

~The right to not be diagnosed with a mental or somatic disorder because a doctor does not understand or believe in Periodic Paralysis~

A somatic disorder is a chronic illness (long-term) with physical symptoms but no known cause is found. It is believed to be fake or not real, but not created 'on purpose' by the individual. This is considered a mental disorder, so this would be what is called, 'all in the mind.' The term 'conversion disorder' is often used for this condition. Most individuals with Periodic Paralysis were and are first diagnosed or mislabeled with this, much to their detriment, before finally obtaining a diagnosis. This is partly why a diagnosis takes an average of twenty years.

This is due to several factors, the first being that Periodic Paralysis looks "fake" to doctors, the second is that sometimes potassium does not shift out of normal ranges and the third being that conversion disorder presents with symptoms that look like Periodic Paralysis according to the standard classification for mental disorders. So rather than diagnosing as Periodic Paralysis, for some reason, the doctors prefer to diagnose with a mental disorder and the doctors who are diagnosing this mental condition, actually have no training to be diagnosing mental disorders.

The question is, "How many diseases or conditions actually exist that can cause intermittent paralysis or muscle weakness based on potassium shifting (even if it is within normal levels)?" Once the tests for those conditions have been completed and ruled out, then a form of Periodic Paralysis is most likely the diagnosis, not mental illness! How many people diagnosed with 'conversion disorder' actually have a form of Periodic Paralysis?

~The right to not be diagnosed with Periodic Paralysis because it is considered "too rare"~

Some doctors have told individuals attempting to obtain a diagnosis for Periodic Paralysis that Periodic Paralysis is "too rare" and could not possibly be what may be wrong with them and causing their symptoms of intermittent muscle weakness and paralysis. The question that needs to be asked of the doctors is, "If not me than whom?" More questions are: "Who are the people who can be diagnosed with a rare condition?" "Do they look different?" "Are they younger?" "Do they have a different color of hair?" "Do they live in a different country?" "Are they shorter or taller?" "Do they have more money?" "Are they male?" "Are they female?" "Could they possibly be sicker?" "Do I need to wait ten more years?"

The truth is, anyone can have a rare genetic disease no matter who he or she is or what he or she looks like. There are more that five thousand rare diseases called orphan diseases, Periodic Paralysis is one of them.

All doctors need to be educated about Periodic Paralysis with up-to-date and correct information. The two or three paragraphs devoted to Periodic Paralysis during medical school is not enough. The information on the Internet is mostly out-dated and faulty at best. Learning about Periodic Paralysis should come from the individuals who have it and experience it everyday. There are many forms of Periodic Paralysis and many variables. Each of us may look different, but each of us has Periodic Paralysis. Periodic Paralysis is not "too rare" for us to have it nor "too rare" for us to be diagnosed with it.

Treatment in the Laboratory

Treatment in the Laboratory

~The right to be treated with respect and dignity by lab technicians~

All medical professionals must treat every patient with Periodic Paralysis, or possible Periodic Paralysis, with respect and dignity just like every other patient with any "more known" medical conditions. This includes the lab technicians with whom we must deal. The lab becomes an issue with individuals with Periodic Paralysis for several reasons.

One of the major features of Periodic Paralysis is the fact that the symptoms are usually related to potassium levels and how they shift or move in error in and out of the cells. The levels, whether low, high or in normal ranges or whether they fluctuate among the three levels is one way to diagnose the type or form of Periodic Paralysis. The potassium level is important for treatment also. This creates the issue of having to be rushed to the lab when paralysis or weakness begins and making sure the blood is drawn in the correct manner and in a timely manner.

Lab technicians do not always understand this protocol when it is presented to them and they want to proceed in ways that will likely taint the outcome of the study. Anger, frustration and rudeness come into play. The patient becomes more stressed making his or her symptoms worse.

Lab technicians need to be trained and educated in how to proceed with an appropriate blood draw for a patient with Periodic Paralysis. The patient has the right to be treated with respect and dignity by lab technicians despite the need for special protocols involving the blood draws for diagnosing and treatment of the condition.

~The right to have blood drawn with no tourniquets~

Studies indicate that using a tourniquet and pumping the hand during a blood draw cause a false potassium result. The reading will indicate a potassium level higher than it is. If a patient actually has low potassium but the results of the testing show low-normal or normal levels due to the tourniquet and hand pumping, the patient may not get the treatment he or she needs, or a diagnosis may be withheld due to normal readings.

Patients have the right to have blood drawn with no tourniquets or hand pumping due to this fact. If potassium is indeed low a patient will need to be treated with potassium in order to bring the levels up. If the potassium is high, the patient will need other treatment to bring the level down. If potassium is within normal levels, no potassium should be given and no other treatment may be necessary other than observing the patient. The potassium levels need to calculated swiftly and correctly.

~The right to have blood drawn as quickly as possible, even if it means going out to the car to draw the blood or to a patient's home~

As discussed previously, timing is important for a blood draw when a patient is in paralysis or experiencing muscle weakness. The blood needs to be drawn right away, because in most cases the shifting happens very quickly. When someone is in paralysis and he or she does not have a potassium reader, it may be difficult for him or her to get out of the car if someone else is driving when an episode begins. At that point lab technicians have been know to go to the patient in the car and take the blood sample. This should always be an option in the case of patients with Periodic Paralysis. Another issue that should be an option is for a patient to have a standing blood draw order in which a lab may be able to have the technician go to the patient's home if it is close enough to get the sample for testing.

~The right to know the potassium level as quickly as possible using an ISTAT or potassium reader~

There are potassium readers, which can be purchased by individuals with Periodic Paralysis in order to monitor the blood potassium levels at home or wherever he or she may be. The problem with these devices is that they are not considered medical devices (however the Food and Drug Administration agrees that the device could easily be deemed as such, but money is the issue for the company who makes them) and insurance will not pay for them. They are very expensive and most families cannot afford them.

These meters should be deemed as medical devices for affordability and immediate treatment issues for families and they should be also available in every lab, ER, hospital and doctor's office.

An ISTAT is another expensive device that measures many vitals, which includes potassium, quickly. These may be available in hospitals and ER's but are not available to individuals with Periodic Paralysis, except by loan from the company, who has only fifty available. Some people waiting to use one have been on a waiting list for several years.

Both devices should be available in the lab and for private use at home and should be paid for by insurance.

~The right for staff to understand that normal potassium levels do not rule out Periodic Paralysis~

Any lab, whether it is private or in a hospital, must train the staff to understand that the results of normal potassium levels do no automatically rule out a diagnosis of Periodic Paralysis. The results only indicate that the normal reading may be a mistake due to using a tourniquet and hand pumping, or that the individual may have Normokalemic Periodic Paralysis, or that the potassium shifted very quickly and was in normal ranges by the time the blood was drawn or that another problem in the cells caused the paralytic attack. A normal potassium level result does not automatically indicate that the patient does not have Periodic Paralysis.

Treatment by Doctors and Medical Professionals

Treatment by Doctors and Medical Professionals

~The right to be treated with respect and dignity by doctors and all medical professionals~

This is the same as in the general rights. The episodes of paralysis or muscle weakness can look "fake" to medical professionals and others. Years of medical testing may reveal no diagnosis. Genetic testing, which is limited and narrow may also be negative for Periodic Paralysis. Due to this, many patients report verbal and mental abuse from their doctors, nurses, technicians and other medical professionals who do not understand the metabolic condition.

Though unbelievable, individuals with Periodic Paralysis, before receiving a diagnosis and some even after, have been lied to; lied about in records; called names; yelled at; watched doctors throw things in anger; hurt while in paralysis when a doctor is trying to prove they are "faking" by scratching, pinching or sticking with pins; refused meds they need; given drugs they do not need; left alone like a naughty child while in paralysis to be punished for bad behavior; scoffed at; laughed at; made to cry; been belittled; told they are "too old" to have the condition and much more. This should never have happened and must not continue to happen in the future.

All medical professionals must treat every patient with Periodic Paralysis, or possible Periodic Paralysis, with respect and dignity just like every other patient with any "more well-known" medical conditions.

~The right for the symptoms of muscle weakness and/or paralysis and other pertinent issues to be taken seriously by doctors~

This is also the same as in the general rights. Medical records indicating decades of odd and severe symptoms, which may appear "fake", medical tests that are always negative, visits to every type of doctor that exists, medications with uncommon side effects, progressive muscle weakness and more are presented to a patient's present doctors or to new doctors who do not know about or understand Periodic Paralysis. These physicians almost immediately begin to view the patient as having mental issues and doubt that a medical issue exists. Words begin to appear in the medical notes with terms like "somatic" or "conversion disorder."

The patient is given drugs for anxiety, depression or psychosis, which causes new symptoms, more paralysis and harmful side effects including the possibility of death. He or she is then dismissed and the symptoms disregarded. He or she is not taken seriously. The patient becomes more ill, and family and friends begin to also dismiss the claims of illness. The patient is expected to continue on with life duties and responsibilities although he or she progressively gets worse. This is wrong and every patient with Periodic Paralysis or the possibility of Periodic Paralysis needs to be taken seriously

~The right for the symptoms of muscle weakness and/or paralysis and other pertinent issues to be thoroughly assessed and treated promptly as needed~

Too often patients with Periodic Paralysis see many doctors and medical professionals and must endure endless medical tests at great cost and much wasted time before receiving a diagnosis. As mentioned before, it takes an average of twenty years; some never getting a diagnosis, as he or she continues to get worse.

When an individual suffering with the symptoms of intermittent muscle weakness or paralysis...partial or full body; heart arrhythmia; heart rate issues...fast or slow; potassium levels...low, high or within normal ranges; blood pressure issues...high or low; breathing issues; low oxygen levels and more, the individual needs to be assessed thoroughly and as quickly as possible and a diagnosis given as soon as possible.

If potassium is found to be low, than potassium may need to be prescribed to stop or minimize the serious symptoms. If potassium levels are high other treatment may be advised. If potassium levels are normal then no treatment may be needed, but information should be given as to how to control and manage the symptoms.

Every patient with Periodic Paralysis has the right to have his or her symptoms of muscle weakness and/or paralysis and other pertinent issues be thoroughly assessed and treated promptly as needed.

~The right to dismiss a doctor for inappropriate care, lack of knowledge of Periodic Paralysis and poor attitude~

For many reasons, as written previously and for others not known, patients with Periodic Paralysis or those with symptoms of Periodic Paralysis who have not received a diagnosis yet, very often report that they are treated very poorly by the doctors they see whether in their offices, in the ER or in a hospital. As mentioned before, though unbelievable, individuals with Periodic Paralysis, before receiving a diagnosis and some even after, have been lied to; lied about in records; called names; yelled at; watched doctors throw things in anger; hurt while in paralysis when a doctor is trying to prove they are "faking" by scratching, pinching or sticking with pins; refused meds they need; given drugs they do not need; left alone like a naughty child while in paralysis to be punished for bad behavior; scoffed at; laughed at; made to cry; been belittled; told they are "too old" to have the condition and much more. This should never have happened and must not continue to happen in the future.

No patient should be treated in such a manner nor should doctors who do not know about or understand Periodic Paralysis or who do not believe in the diagnosis be allowed to continue with such behavior. A patient has the right to fire or remove a doctor from his or her care. He or she has the right to dismiss a doctor for inappropriate care, lack of knowledge of Periodic Paralysis and poor attitude.

~The right to refuse any and all drugs prescribed by a doctor; to include IV's and anesthesia~

Periodic Paralysis is a medical condition like no other. There is only one drug or medication (which has just been approved by the FDA) approved by the FDA to treat it. There are a few 'off-label' drugs (created for other uses), however, that are prescribed and used for a few forms of the mineral metabolic disorder. For most of the mutations, however, these drugs are harmful, can cause serious side effects and over long time use can cause even more serious side effects and even death.

Due to the nature of a mineral metabolic disorder, any and all drugs, including over-the-counter drugs, can cause serious symptoms and trigger episodes of paralysis, heart arrhythmia and even death. This includes IV's, especially saline (sodium) and glucose (sugar) IV's, anesthesia, all forms, including topical forms and even contrast dyes in MRI's. These should be avoided and an individual with Periodic Paralysis or suspected Periodic Paralysis has the right to refuse them and must refuse them from their doctors, in an ambulance, in the ER and in a hospital.

If an IV must be administered, mannitol, extremely diluted, may be used with great care. If a patient must attempt to take a drug or medication he or she should begin with an amount at about ¼ of what a normal person may use and should be observed very closely.

~The right for clear, concise and truthful medical notes and records to be written by the doctors and other medical professionals~

As already stated, patients with Periodic Paralysis or those with symptoms of Periodic Paralysis who have not received a diagnosis yet, very often report that they are treated very poorly by the doctors they see whether in their offices, in the ER or in a hospital. And as mentioned before, though unbelievable, individuals with Periodic Paralysis, before receiving a diagnosis and some even after, have been "lied to;" "lied about" in medical records and office notes.

Patients with Periodic Paralysis report obtaining their medical records from the doctors, ER visits, hospital stays, testing and more. Upon reading through them many blatant lies were discovered. For instance, found was, "patient refused to raise her leg when asked" rather than the truth, "patient could not raise her leg when asked." Another patient's record stated she was "working on her third marriage" when the truth of the matter is, she has been married for over thirty years in this third marriage. One individual had to be carried out of the hospital by her husband after lapsing into paralysis because the doctor gave her a drug, after the patient and her husband told him not to. The record stated that the drug helped the patient and she and her husband left after an exit meeting. There was no exit meeting and the drug caused more paralysis and other serious symptoms. In another case, some records indicated that testing resulted in positive results for Periodic Paralysis, but the patient was told that testing was negative.

Lying by doctors and medical professionals must stop.

~The right to read and receive copies of all medical records and the right to challenge, add to and to change their content if not accurate~

In the National Patient's Bills of Rights, regarding privacy and confidentiality, every patient has the 'right to copy and read all medical records and to change anything that is incorrect or not relevant and to add to records which are not complete.' So, every patient with Periodic Paralysis has the same right to receive copies of all medical records and the right to challenge what is written in them. If information is missing whether it is a simple mistake or done on purpose, it needs to be added. If discrepancies, misconceptions and lies are discovered, these need to be challenged and changed. It should also be reported. No one has a right to lie about another person. No doctor should have the right to lie about a patient.

~The right to complain and make appeals about any doctor or medical care provider, regarding waiting time, actions or non-actions and adequacy of services~

Complaining and making appeals about any medical care provider, regarding waiting time, actions or non-actions and adequacy of services or facilities is also listed in the National Patient's Bills of Rights. If a doctor or medical care provider is in any way creating problems for a patient with Periodic Paralysis regarding time issues, causing harm in some manner by what he or she is doing or not doing or is not adequately treating him or her, then the doctor needs to be reported. Complaints need to and must be filed.

~The right to be referred to a doctor who understands Periodic Paralysis~

As explained previously, most doctors do not know about or understand the different forms of Periodic Paralysis. There are some who do know a little about it but most of them are using erroneous and out-dated information for diagnosing (or not diagnosing) and treating the patients. 'Specialist' do exist, but most of them a purists; they know about the forms of Periodic Paralysis, which are 'cut and dried.' If someone's potassium is low during periods of intermittent paralysis or weakness then Hypokalemic Periodic Paralysis can be easily diagnosed as long as no others conditions coexist. If someone's potassium is high during periods of intermittent paralysis or weakness then Hyperkalemic Periodic Paralysis can be easily diagnosed as long as no others conditions coexist. If genetic testing reveals a known mutation for any of the known forms, then a diagnosis is easily made.

However, many of the individuals with Periodic Paralysis have atypical symptoms and characteristics and other autoimmune or mitochondrial conditions, which coexist. About fifty percent of individuals do not have a known mutation that has yet been discovered and genetic testing is biased and narrow. The 'specialists' do not want to, nor do they, diagnose these individuals.

Neurologists, who see most patients with this condition, do not understand that it is a mineral metabolic disorder not a neurological disorder. This creates issues for diagnosing and treatment.

Patients need to be referred to or be able to seek out doctors who do understand it and are willing to work with them for diagnosing and treatment.

Treatment in the ER and Hospital

Treatment in the ER and Hospital

~The right to be treated with respect and dignity by doctors and medical professionals~

This is the same as in the general rights and for treatment by doctors and the medical professionals. In the emergency room (ER) the episodes of paralysis or muscle weakness can appear "fake." If years of medical testing reveal no diagnosis and genetic testing, which is limited and narrow, is negative for Periodic Paralysis, many patients report verbal and mental abuse from their doctors, nurses, technicians and other medical professionals who do not understand the metabolic condition when they are seen in the ER.

As written previously, these individuals with Periodic Paralysis, before receiving a diagnosis and some even after, in the ER have been lied to; lied about in records; called names; yelled at; watched doctors throw things in anger; hurt while in paralysis when a doctor is trying to prove they are "faking" by scratching, pinching or sticking with pins; refused meds they need; given drugs they do not need; left alone like a naughty child while in paralysis to be punished for bad behavior; scoffed at; laughed at; made to cry; been belittled; told they are "too old" to have the condition and much more. This should never happen and must not continue to happen in the future.

All medical professionals in the ER must treat every patient with Periodic Paralysis, or possible Periodic Paralysis, with respect and dignity just like every other patient with any "more well-known" medical conditions.

~The right to be seen quickly~

Too often patients with Periodic Paralysis are rushed to the ER in an ambulance only to be left alone and much time may pass before they are seen, assessed or treated. Due to the nature of the seriousness of the episodes, one needs to be observed and assessed very quickly. Potassium levels need to be tested as soon as possible.

When an individual suffering with the symptoms of intermittent muscle weakness or paralysis...partial or full body; heart arrhythmia; heart rate issues...fast or slow; potassium levels...low, high or within normal ranges; blood pressure issues...high or low; breathing issues; low oxygen levels, choking and more, the individual needs to be assessed thoroughly and quickly. Patients may and have been known to die in severe episodes from cardiac and/or respiratory arrest.

If potassium is found to be low, than potassium may need to be administered right away to stop the serious symptoms. If potassium levels are high other treatment may be needed. If potassium levels are normal then no treatment may be needed, but the patient should never be left alone and must be observed for all of the issues above.

If the patient, family members or caregivers have specific information or treatment guidelines the medical team must follow them.

If the patient does not have a diagnosis, the ER doctor may make the diagnosis based on the obvious symptoms and results of the testing and assessments and results of the treatment.

Every patient with Periodic Paralysis in the ER has the right to be seen immediately and to have his or her symptoms of muscle weakness and/or paralysis and other pertinent issues assessed and treated.

~The right to be comfortable and safe~

During episodes of paralysis or muscle weakness, a patient with Periodic Paralysis is very weak or totally incapacitated and extremely vulnerable. If in full-body paralysis, the patient is totally unable to move in any way, the eyes are closed, the mouth is unable to speak, the heart may be racing or too slow and beating erratically, blood pressure may be high or low, oxygen may be low, choking may occur and pain may be an issue. He or she can hear everything being said and knows what is happening. Episodes of weakness may be full-body or partial. No matter how the episode is manifested, it is very frightening for the patient and the loved ones or caregivers who may be with him or her.

The patient may need to be positioned on their side or with their head elevated to avoid choking and to aid with breathing. He or she needs to be made comfortable, since movement in any way for them may be impossible. It is important to make sure they are not too cold or too hot since either can trigger more paralysis.

Every patient with Periodic Paralysis or symptoms of Periodic Paralysis needs to be made comfortable and kept safe.

~The right to be accompanied and observed constantly by medical staff when in a paralytic episode~

Because a patient with Periodic Paralysis is very weak or totally incapacitated and extremely vulnerable he or she should never be left alone. Due to the serious symptoms that accompany each paralytic episode, he or she must be constantly observed. The medical professionals must monitor one's heart, blood pressure, oxygen, potassium, breathing, temperature, positioning and more.

~The right for the doctors and medical professionals to listen to the patient (if possible), family members or caregivers on instruction for care~

Periodic Paralysis is a condition in which most medical professionals know very little, as discussed previously. Therefore most patients with it or who suspect they have it do a great deal of research. The patient and loved ones usually know what works the best such as positioning, blood draws without a tourniquet or potassium and the things that they should avoid such as IV's and drugs. This information is related to the staff in the ambulance and upon arrival in the ER to keep the patient safe and comfortable and hopefully as stress-free as possible.

Unfortunately, patients report that doctors and medical professionals ignore this important information, refuse to listen or argue with them or their family members or caregivers. This can and does create stress for the patient and loved ones and the patient may be harmed if the proper instructions are not followed. Every patient with Periodic Paralysis or who suspects he or she may have it, has the right to have the doctors and medical professionals listen to him or her (if possible), family members or caregivers on instruction for care.

~The right for the doctors and medical professionals to read information provided by the patient, family members or caregivers on how to care for the patient~

As stated before, Periodic Paralysis is a condition in which most medical professionals know very little. Therefore most patients and family members with it or who suspect they have it do a great deal of research. The latest information is gathered and collected in some manner to be shared in an emergency. The personal information about what works best for him or her is also included. Some carry notebooks, some use USB sticks or computer disks, some have bracelets with information, some wear information in pouches around their necks and some may carry one or two of the books written about it. Some may even go to the hospital in the area and have this information copied and in the system in case they end up in the ER.

Unfortunately, patients report that doctors and medical professionals ignore this important information, refuse to read it and argue with them or their family members or caregivers. This can and does create stress for the patient and loved ones and the patient may be harmed if the proper instructions are not followed. Every patient with Periodic Paralysis, or who suspects he or she may have it, has the right to have the doctors and medical professionals read information provided by the patient, family members or caregivers on how to care for the condition.

~The right for all doctors and medical professionals to follow the specific instructions provided to include proper positioning, no IV's, no drugs and more, as necessary~

The doctors and medical professionals who see patients with Periodic Paralysis or with symptoms that appear to be Periodic Paralysis have the duty to listen to the patient (if possible), his or her family members or caregivers. They have the duty to read information provided by the patient, family members or caregivers on how to care for the patient and they have the duty to follow the specific instructions provided, to include proper positioning, blood draws without tourniquets, no IV's, no drugs and much more, as necessary.

The patient has the right to be safe and comfortable and to be treated with respect and dignity. He or she has the right to not be harmed by the medical professionals and doctors he or she sees in the ambulance, emergency room or hospital.

~The right for blood to be drawn with no tourniquets for potassium levels which may indicate potassium levels that may be low, high or within normal ranges~

To reiterate: Studies indicate that using a tourniquet and pumping the hand during a blood draw cause a false potassium result. The reading will indicate a potassium level higher than it is. If a patient actually has low potassium but the results of the testing show low-normal or normal levels due to the tourniquet and hand pumping, the patient may not get the treatment he or she needs, or a diagnosis may be withheld due to normal readings.

Patients have the right to have blood drawn with no tourniquets or hand pumping due to this fact. If potassium is indeed low, a patient will need to be treated with potassium in order to bring the levels up. If the potassium is high, the patient will need other treatment to bring the level down. If potassium is within normal levels, no potassium should be given and no other treatment may be necessary other than observing the patient. The levels need to be measured swiftly and correctly.

~The right for blood to be drawn as quickly as possible preferably using a potassium reader or ISTAT for instant results which may indicate potassium levels that may be low, high or within normal ranges~

As previously mentioned, timing is important for a blood draw when a patient is in paralysis or experiencing muscle weakness. The blood needs to be drawn right away, because in most cases the shifting happens very quickly. This is an important issue in the ER.

Potassium readers, which measure potassium levels and ISTAT's, which measure many vitals, including potassium quickly, should be available in hospitals and ER's for instant results.

~The right for the symptoms of muscle weakness and/or paralysis, and other pertinent issues to be thoroughly assessed~

Too often patients with Periodic Paralysis are rushed to the ER to be left alone and much time may pass before they are seen, assessed or treated. Due to the nature of the seriousness of the episodes, one needs to be observed and assessed in the ER very quickly. Potassium levels need to be tested as soon as possible.

When an individual suffering with the symptoms of intermittent muscle weakness or paralysis...partial or full body; heart arrhythmia; heart rate issues...fast or slow; potassium levels...low, high or within normal ranges; blood pressure issues...high or low; breathing issues; low oxygen levels and more, the individual needs to be assessed thoroughly and quickly.

If potassium is found to be low, than potassium may need to be administered right away to stop the serious symptoms. If potassium levels are high other treatment may be needed. If potassium levels are normal then no treatment may be needed, but the patient should never be left alone and must be observed for all of the issues above.

If the patient, family members or caregivers have specific information or treatment guidelines the medical team must follow them.

If the patient does not have a diagnosis, the ER doctor may make the diagnosis based on the obvious symptoms and results of the testing and assessments and results of the treatment.

Every patient with Periodic Paralysis has the right to have his or her symptoms of muscle weakness and/or paralysis and other pertinent issues to be thoroughly assessed and treated promptly.

~The right for the symptoms of muscle weakness and/or paralysis and others as pertinent to be taken seriously by the doctors and medical care professionals~

As written earlier: This is the same as in the general rights. Medical records indicating decades of odd and severe symptoms, which may appear "fake", medical tests that are always negative, visits to every type of doctor which exists, medications with uncommon side effects, progressive muscle weakness and more are presented to a patient's present doctors or to new doctors who do not know about or understand Periodic Paralysis and especially those in the emergency room, these physicians almost immediately begin to view the patient as having mental issues and doubt that a medical issue exists. Words begin to appear in the medical notes with terms like "somatic," "pseudo-seizures" or "conversion disorder."

The patient is given drugs for anxiety, depression or psychosis, which causes new symptoms, more paralysis and harmful side effects including the possibility of death. He or she is then dismissed and the symptoms disregarded. He or she is not taken seriously. The patient becomes more ill, and family and friends begin to also dismiss the claims of illness. The patient is expected to continue on with life duties and responsibilities though he or she progressively gets worse. This is wrong and every patient with Periodic Paralysis or the possibility of Periodic Paralysis needs to be taken seriously and treated appropriately, especially in the emergency room.

~The right to be observed for choking, heart arrhythmia, fluctuations in blood pressure, and heart rate, breathing issues, low oxygen levels and others as pertinent~

Written previously: Too often patients with Periodic Paralysis are rushed to the ER in an ambulance only to be left alone and much time may pass before they are seen, assessed or treated. Due to the nature of the seriousness of the episodes, one needs to be observed and assessed very quickly. Potassium levels need to be tested as soon as possible.

When an individual is suffering with the symptoms of intermittent muscle weakness or paralysis...partial or full body; heart arrhythmia; heart rate issues...fast or slow; potassium levels...low, high or within normal ranges; blood pressure issues...high or low; breathing issues; low oxygen levels, choking and more, he or she needs to be assessed thoroughly and quickly. Patients may, and have been known to, die in severe episodes from cardiac and/or respiratory arrest.

For this reason, patients with Periodic Paralysis or possible Periodic Paralysis, have the right to be observed for choking, heart arrhythmia, fluctuations in blood pressure, and heart rate, breathing issues, low oxygen levels and others as pertinent for possible emergency treatment and life-saving procedures.

~The right to not be harmed during paralysis by doctors or other medical professionals attempting to prove "faking" by pinching, scratching, burning or sticking with pins or needles~

Previously stated: The episodes of paralysis or muscle weakness can look "fake" to medical professionals and others in the emergency room. Due to this, many patients report verbal and mental abuse from their doctors, nurses, technicians and other medical professionals who do not understand the metabolic condition, especially in the ER.

Though unbelievable, individuals with Periodic Paralysis, before receiving a diagnosis and some even after, are hurt while in paralysis when a doctor is trying to prove they are "faking" by scratching, pinching or sticking with pins or other sharp articles as they lay on a gurney or bed, unable to defend themselves or move in any way, but very much aware of the pain and conversation of the medical staff.

All medical professionals must treat every patient with Periodic Paralysis, or possible Periodic Paralysis, with respect and dignity just like every other patient with any "more known" medical conditions.

~The right to be treated for choking, heart arrhythmia, fluctuations in blood pressure, and heart rate, breathing issues, low oxygen levels as pertinent~

As stated above: Too often patients with Periodic Paralysis are rushed to the ER in an ambulance only to be left alone and much time may pass before they are seen, assessed or treated. Due to the nature of the seriousness of the episodes, one needs to be observed and assessed very quickly. Potassium levels need to be tested as soon as possible.

When an individual is suffering with the symptoms of intermittent muscle weakness or paralysis...partial or full body; heart arrhythmia; heart rate issues...fast or slow; potassium levels...low, high or within normal ranges; blood pressure issues...high or low; breathing issues; low oxygen levels, choking and more, he or she needs to be assessed thoroughly and quickly. Patients may, and have been known to, die in severe episodes from cardiac and/or respiratory arrest.

If potassium is found to be low, than potassium may need to be administered right away to stop the serious symptoms. If potassium levels are high other treatment may be needed. If potassium levels are normal then no treatment may be needed, but the patient should never be left alone and must be observed for all of the issues above.

If the patient, family members or caregivers have specific information or treatment guidelines the medical team must follow them.

If the patient does not have a diagnosis, the ER doctor may make the diagnosis based on the obvious symptoms and results of the testing and assessments and results of the treatment.

~The right to refuse IV's, drugs, medications and anesthesia, which may be harmful or deadly~

In an ambulance and in the emergency room the first line of assistance usually given to a patient is being placed on an IV. This can create great harm and even death to an individual with Periodic Paralysis.

Periodic Paralysis is a medical condition like no other, as described previously. There is only one drug or medication (which has just been approved by the FDA) approved by the FDA to treat it. There are a few 'off-label' drugs (created for other uses), however, that are prescribed and used for a few forms of the mineral metabolic disorder. For most of the mutations, however, these drugs are harmful, can cause serious side effects and over long time use can cause even more serious side effects and even death.

Due to the nature of a mineral metabolic disorder, any and all drugs, including over-the-counter drugs, can cause serious symptoms and trigger episodes of paralysis, heart arrhythmia and even death. This includes IV's, especially saline (sodium) and glucose (sugar) IV's, anesthesia, all forms, including topical forms and even contrasts in MRI's. These should be avoided and an individual with Periodic Paralysis or suspected Periodic Paralysis has the right to refuse them and must refuse them from their doctors, in an ambulance, in the ER and in a hospital.

If an IV must be administered, mannitol, extremely diluted, may be used with great care. If a patient must attempt to take a drug or medication he or she should begin with an amount at about ¼ of what a normal person may use.

~The right to refuse provocative testing for the reason of diagnosing Periodic Paralysis~

As explained before, it was discovered some time back that due to the nature of a mineral metabolic disorder, there were things that could trigger the symptoms of muscle weakness and paralysis. These triggers, depending on the particular form of Periodic Paralysis, include but are not limited to, most drugs, IV's (glucose and saline) anesthesia, salt, sugar, potassium, gluten, food fillers and dyes, sleep, exercise, cold, heat and stress.

Doctors in the emergency rooms, not understanding the serious implications of being in a paralytic episode including dangerous heart arrhythmia (even possibly long QT heart beats), dangerous heart rate and blood pressure fluctuations, low oxygen levels, choking, breathing cessation, cardiac and respiratory arrest and possible death; decided that in order to prove or disprove the existence of the condition, could "provoke" the symptoms and paralysis by putting a patient on an IV of glucose and then when the symptoms begin, quickly give them potassium to stop it.

Because some forms of Periodic Paralysis are just the opposite or react in different ways, some of these patients died. Provoking an attack of paralysis is NEVER to be done. It is far too risky and can end in death.

Any and every patient with Periodic Paralysis has the right to refuse the provocation of his or her symptoms by a doctor or other medical care professionals in the emergency room or the hospital.

~The right to call in a hospitalist, or other specialists who may know about Periodic Paralysis as needed~

Most hospitals have a specialized physician called a hospitalist. Their main focus is caring for hospitalized patients. They are usually in a leadership role in the hospital and are involved in the care of patients, teaching the staff and research. For this reason, a hospitalist may need to be called in to guide the emergency room staff or hospital staff on how to treat a patient with Periodic Paralysis and teach the staff at the same time for future patients with the condition or if the patient may need to return for care. If the hospitalist does not know about Periodic Paralysis, it would be his or her job and responsibility to learn about all aspects of it and then teach the staff to care appropriately for the patient.

So, if a doctor in the emergency room does not know about Periodic Paralysis or how to treat a patient with Periodic Paralysis, the patient and his or her family or caregiver has the right to request a hospitalist, or other specialists who may know about Periodic Paralysis for treatment and diagnosis.

~The right to call in a social worker or patient advocate as needed~

As previously explained, individuals with Periodic Paralysis and their family members are often treated very poorly when they arrive in the ER, due to the nature of the symptoms and the difficulty in diagnosing the condition. Calling in a hospital social worker or patient advocate may be necessary in order to gain some support and options for care and treatment and to assist with conflict which may arise between the patient and the medical professionals.

Most hospitals hire patient advocates to assist the patients who are receiving care. Their main job is to handle the complaints made by patients regarding their care and the medical professionals providing that care. Social workers assess the psychological and social functioning of patients and families and intervene as necessary. They work in conjunction with the medical professionals on a patient's team, including doctors, nurses and therapists.

Hopefully, the hospitalists, social workers and patient advocates will be able to assist the patients with Periodic Paralysis and their families and caregivers to communicate better with the medical team in order to get the proper treatment required in the best way possible in a stress-free environment.

~The right to dismiss a doctor or other medical professional for inappropriate care, lack of knowledge of Periodic Paralysis and poor attitude~

As previously written and for others not known, patients with Periodic Paralysis or those with symptoms of Periodic Paralysis who have not yet received a diagnosis, very often report that they are treated very poorly by the doctors they see in the ER or hospital. As mentioned before, these individuals with Periodic Paralysis, before receiving a diagnosis and some even after, have been lied to; lied about in records; called names; yelled at; watched doctors throw things in anger; hurt while in paralysis when a doctor is trying to prove they are "faking" by scratching, pinching or sticking with pins; refused meds they need; given drugs they do not need; left alone like a naughty child while in paralysis to be punished for bad behavior; scoffed at; laughed at; made to cry; been belittled; told they are "too old" to have the condition and much more. This should never have happened and must not continue to happen in the future.

No patient in an emergency room or hospital should be treated in such a manner nor should doctors who do not know about or understand Periodic Paralysis or who do not believe in the diagnosis be allowed to continue with such behavior. A patient in the ER has the right to fire or remove a doctor from his or her care. He or she has the right to dismiss a doctor for inappropriate care, lack of knowledge of Periodic Paralysis and poor attitude.

~The right for clear, concise and truthful medical notes and records to be written by the doctors and other medical professionals~

It is now known and has been discussed previously that patients with Periodic Paralysis or those with symptoms of Periodic Paralysis who have not yet received a diagnosis, very often report doctors treat them very poorly, especially in the ER or in a hospital. It is common to be "lied to" and "lied about" in the ER and hospital records.

Patients with Periodic Paralysis report obtaining their medical records from emergency room visits, hospital stays and testing and upon reading through them, many out-right lies were discovered. For instance, found was, "patient refused to raise her leg when asked" rather than the truth, "patient could not raise her leg when asked." Another patient's record stated that she was "working on her third marriage" when the truth of the matter is, she has been married for over thirty years in this third marriage. One individual had to be carried out of the hospital by her husband after slipping into paralysis because the doctor gave her a drug, after the patient and her husband told him not to. The record stated that the drug helped the patient and she and her husband left after an exit meeting. There was no exit meeting and the drug created more paralysis and other serious symptoms. In another case, some records indicated that testing resulted in positive results for Periodic Paralysis, but the patients were told the testing results were negative.

Lying by doctors and medical professionals must stop. Everyone with Periodic Paralysis has the right for clear, concise and truthful medical notes and records to be written by the doctors and other medical professionals.

~The right to read and receive copies of all medical records and the right to challenge, add to and to change the content if not accurate~

In the National Patient's Bills of Rights, regarding privacy and confidentiality, every patient has the 'right to copy and read all medical records and to change anything that is incorrect or not relevant and to add to records which are not complete.' So, every patient with Periodic Paralysis has the same right to receive copies of all medical records written in the emergency room or the hospital and the right to challenge what is written in them. If information is missing whether it is a simple mistake or done on purpose, it needs to be added. If discrepancies, misconceptions and lies are discovered, these need to be challenged and changed. It should also be reported. No one has a right to lie about another person. No doctor or other medical professional should have the right to lie about a patient in the emergency room or the hospital.

~The right to complain and make appeals about any doctor or medical care provider, regarding waiting time, actions or non-actions and adequacy of services~

Complaining and making appeals about any doctor or medical care provider, regarding waiting time, actions or non-actions and adequacy of services or facilities is also listed in the National Patient's Bills of Rights. If a doctor or medical care provider has in any way created problems for a patient with Periodic Paralysis regarding time issues, causing harm in some manner by what he or she is doing or not doing or is not adequately treating him or her, then the doctor or medical professional must be reported. Complaints need to be and must be filed.

Research and Awareness

Research and Awareness

~The right to increasing awareness of Periodic Paralysis among populations, doctors and governments~

Awareness is a sense of understanding, knowing, recognition or mindfulness of something. At this time, among most people in the world, doctors, medical professionals and government entities, the term Periodic Paralysis has no meaning. It is not recognized, known about or understood by those in authority who should be aware of it. This needs to be changed worldwide.

Too many individuals are suffering needlessly and even dying due to under-recognition, under-diagnosis and misdiagnosis. This has to stop. Some form of funding should be available to aid those who know about and understand the condition to bring about awareness of it to people in all over the world, medical professionals who should be able to recognize, diagnose and treat it and to governments for research.

~The right to "put a face" to Periodic Paralysis as in other known diseases and medical conditions~

When the terms multiple sclerosis, muscular dystrophy, ALS (Lou Gehrig's disease), cancer or leukemia are heard someone automatically visualizes an individual whose health is compromised, probably in some pain, maybe in a wheelchair and unable to go about normal daily duties, unaided. The futures of these individuals are uncertain. Most people are moved to sadness and concern for those individuals. Family, friends, churches, and even entire neighborhoods and communities readily offer help and support.

When someone suffering the effects of the cruel condition of Periodic Paralysis mentions the term 'Periodic Paralysis' blank stares and lack of understanding are the norm. Very few people on earth have heard of it or know about it. This needs to be changed.

When the words "Periodic Paralysis" are heard everyone should instantly visualize an individual becoming suddenly totally paralyzed, unable to walk or talk and in fear because his or her heart is racing and beating irregularly, blood pressure is dangerously high or low, breathing is difficult and may stop, oxygen may be very low, choking may occur, and he or she may die during the episode from a heart arrhythmia and/or respiratory or cardiac arrest. He or she looks asleep or unconscious, but can hear everything going on, but cannot say a word. The individual is vulnerable and at the mercy of others and 'totally alone in the dark.' Over time, gradual, permanent muscle weakness sets in and the person becomes disabled. The future of these individuals is as uncertain as in the other conditions.

~The right for all medical professionals to be educated about all aspects of Periodic Paralysis including all forms, the symptoms for each and the appropriate treatment for each~

As explained earlier, it takes nearly a decade of graduate school to become a doctor. During those years of training, Periodic Paralysis is mentioned in one or two paragraphs and in those paragraphs it is described as so rare that a doctor will never see a patient with it in his or her lifetime or years of practice. This is a serious disservice to those of us who have the condition.

As it turns out Periodic Paralysis is not all that "rare," but rather it is under-recognized and under-diagnosed and mis-diagnosed. As stated before, it takes an average of twenty years for an individual to receive a diagnosis. Many die before they ever receive a diagnosis. This is unconscionable and unnecessary. This would not be the case if all medical professionals understood Periodic Paralysis and knew how to recognize this condition.

More education and training is needed for students in medical school and for all other medical professionals including nurses, EMT's, paramedics, social workers, teachers, lab technicians and more. Periodic Paralysis needs to be as commonly understood as other medical conditions such as multiple sclerosis, muscular dystrophy, fibromyalgia, heart disease, diabetes, and Lou Gehrig's disease.

For those with Periodic Paralysis, health is compromised, many are in pain, wheelchairs may be needed and living a normal life unaided is impossible. The future for these individuals is uncertain.

Doctors need to understand this and family, friends, churches, neighborhoods and communities need to readily offer help, understanding and support.

~The right to funding for research of all aspects of Periodic Paralysis including but not limited to diagnosis and treatment~

Periodic Paralysis should be as easily recognized as all of the well-known and more common serious medical conditions. The individuals with this condition have seriously compromised health and live in pain and fear, usually end up in a wheelchair, and are unable to go about normal daily duties, unaided. The futures of these individuals are as uncertain as those with multiple sclerosis, muscular dystrophy, ALS, cancer or leukemia.

Without a diagnosis and treatment, it is not uncommon for friends to stop visiting, family members become doubtful and consider a mental disorder (If doctors do not believe it, why would the family members?) The ability to work is compromised. There is a loss of jobs, careers and income. Losing one's home, marriage and family may occur. Becoming totally dependent on others follows. There is a loss of the ability to do favorite hobbies and activities. One loses hope as well as their dreams and desires.

This is unconscionable and unnecessary. Individuals with Periodic Paralysis deserve and need answers, help, respect, acknowledgement and care, as does anyone else with a more common condition. Funding needs to be available for providing these things and for researching all aspects of Periodic Paralysis, including but not limited to diagnosis, treatment, genetics, equipment, medication, medical devices and equipment. It should also be available for training medical professionals and for awareness of this cruel condition.

Insurance

Insurance

~The right for all forms of Periodic Paralysis to be recognized as disabling conditions by insurance companies~

Periodic Paralysis is not a neuromuscular, mitochondrial or autoimmune disease nor is it a muscular dystrophy. It is a rare condition like no other, called an ion channelopathy also called a mineral metabolic disorder. Ion channelopathies were first recognized in 1971 and a form of Periodic Paralysis was the first to be discovered. An ion channelopathy is a dysfunction of an ion channel, which is like a microscopic tunnel in the cells of muscles. They regulate contraction and relaxation of the muscle.

Unfortunately, ion channelopathies are not usually categorized nor listed in medical writing or studies as metabolic disorders. This poses a problem for recognition, diagnosis and treatment by physicians and other medical professionals and poses a problem for insurance purposes.

Upon seeing a doctor, a diagnosis is assigned or reasons for that visit is noted on a form, in triplicate, used for billing insurance. The form has catagorized diseases or diagnoses listed with a number assigned to each. These names and numbers are used worldwide in a system called the ICD-10 Codes Registry. Periodic Paralysis is the number: G723 (G72.3) and is categorized as a disease of the nervous system and sub-categorized as a neuromuscular disease. This is not correct.

This needs to be changed and recognized to avoid more confusion. Periodic Paralysis needs to be listed as what it is; a disabling mineral metabolic disorder or ion channelopathy.

~The right for potassium readers to be deemed as medical devices and paid for by insurance companies~

Pharmaceuticals are not the answer for treatment of Periodic Paralysis. Rather than medications and drugs, individuals with Periodic Paralysis must measure potassium in the body in order to help monitor and relieve symptoms and stay alive by avoiding paralytic episodes. This can be done with a device called a potassium meter or reader. The hand-held devices measure the potassium levels easily and quickly at home or wherever needed. The problem with them is that they are not considered medical devices (however the Food and Drug Administration agrees that the device could easily be deemed as such, but money is the issue for the company who makes them) and insurance will not pay for them. They are very expensive (about $350.00 each) and most families cannot afford them thus making the monitoring of symptoms very difficult and leaving individuals at risk.

These meters should be deemed as medical devices for affordability and immediate treatment issues for families and they should be also available in every lab, ER, hospital and doctor's office.

~The right to have ISTAT devices for monitoring vitals for all Periodic Paralysis patients and to have them paid for by insurance companies~

An ISTAT is an easy to use hand-held medical device that uses blood to measure many different vitals in real-time to include all electrolytes, heart markers, gases, chemistries and blood issues. These measurements are important because those with Periodic Paralysis, especially when in an episode of paralysis or muscle weakness, are affected in each of these areas. Knowledge of these measurements can aid in treatment. Maintaining a balance in these areas is also important to avoid the episodes, so daily use of the small apparatus can be very important. Unfortunately, ISTAT's are used in hospitals, but are not available for home use.

When in a paralytic episode, an individual needs to have his or her vital signs monitored constantly. It is not necessary to go to the hospital each time as long a friend, family member or caregiver is near and observing the symptoms. This can be done with potassium readers, finger oximeters, blood pressure cuffs, glucose meters, and thermometers, but much remains unanswered and unknown. The ISTAT will provide the necessary information for proper treatment. The ISTAT devices should be available and prescribed for home use in order to monitor vital signs for all Periodic Paralysis patients and insurance companies should pay for the devices.

~The right for the special natural and organic diet and supplementation that must be followed by patients with Periodic Paralysis to be paid for in part by insurance companies~

Most individuals must control the serious symptoms of Periodic Paralysis by natural means. This includes discovering and avoiding all known triggers, following a special diet and using natural and organic supplements.

Most drugs, medications and pharmaceuticals are known and serious triggers for the episodes of paralysis and can even cause death. They must be avoided.

The diet consists of eating organic and natural foods, avoiding all processed foods and foods with fillers or dyes. Most individuals also need to avoid gluten, sugar, salt, fat and carbohydrates. Food and water with antibiotics and pesticides must also be avoided. This diet is very expensive and not always affordable for many patients with this condition.

Unfortunately, this may be the only way for many to avoid the disabling symptoms, muscle weakness and paralysis and provide some quality of life to the patient. Therefore, it seems only right that medical insurance companies pays for, either in full or in part, the food necessary to treat and manage the cruel symptoms of Periodic Paralysis and maintain some quality of life.

Conclusion

It is our greatest hope and desire that this booklet, *A Bill Of Rights for Periodic Paralysis Patients,* can be a tool or an instrument that will bring awareness to the rare and disabling mineral metabolic disorder known as Periodic Paralysis. We hope that those who read it will be educated in all aspects of Periodic Paralysis, including but not limited to the symptoms, the diagnosis and the treatment.

We also hope to bring awareness of the plight of the courageous individuals who suffer from the unrelenting affects of the cruel condition, daily. We hope that through this awareness, the wrongs that they experience at the hands of the doctors and medical professionals, with whom they must rely upon, will be made right and corrected.

We hope also, that this knowledge will empower all individuals with Periodic Paralysis to support and defend themselves in dealing with all medical professionals, in all situations, by knowing and understanding their medical rights. This includes their general rights, diagnosis, treatment in labs, treatment by doctors and treatment in the emergency room and the areas of research, awareness and insurance.

Finally, we hope the doctors, medical professionals and all others who may have occasion to deal with Periodic Paralysis patients in some manner, to include but not limited to; insurance companies, pharmaceutical companies, adaptive equipment companies, medical device companies and genetic research laboratories; will recognize themselves in this book and begin to make changes in the manner with which they deal with individuals with all forms of Periodic Paralysis, or the part they play in their lives, to insure correct and proper recognition, diagnosis, treatment, care and follow-up.

For more information about Periodic Paralysis:
The following are the services and features of our PPN forum:

PPN Website: www.periodicparalysisnetwork.com

PPN Books:
Living With Periodic Paralysis: The Mystery Unraveled
https://www.createspace.com/4111713

The Periodic Paralysis Guide And Workbook: Be The Best You Can Be Naturally
https://www.createspace.com/4326356

(Also found on our website)
http://www.periodicparalysisnetwork.com/books.htm

PPN Blog: http://livingwithperiodicparalysis.blogspot.com/

PPN Support, Education and Advocacy Group:
https://www.facebook.com/groups/periodicparalysisnetworksupportgroup/

PPN Book Discussion Group:
https://www.facebook.com/groups/periodicparalysisnetwork/

PPN Genealogy Discussion Group:
https://www.facebook.com/groups/580168915344191/

PPNI Genetics Discussion and Research Group.
https://www.facebook.com/groups/1574048096186578/

The PPN Learning Center and Workshop:
https://www.facebook.com/groups/1416848568618404/

PPN Website Facebook Page:
https://www.facebook.com/PeriodicParalysisNetwork

PPN Author's Page:
https://www.facebook.com/SusanQKnittleHunterauthor

Email: sqknittle@gmail.com

Fund raisers:
GoFundMe: http://www.gofundme.com/ftnr50
Bravelets: https://www.bravelets.com/bravepage/alone-in-the-dark-periodic-paralysis

 Please check out our PPN Members World Map:
http://www.multiplottr.com/?map_id=55083

About the Authors

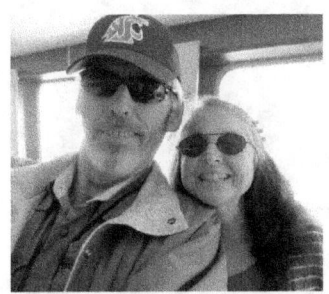 Calvin and Susan Q. Knittle-Hunter are the co-creators, co-founders and co-directors of the Periodic Paralysis Network, Inc. (PPNI), an independent, educational corporation, designed to provide support, education and advocacy to individuals with Periodic Paralysis (PP).

Susan, the Managing Director of PPNI, earned B.S. degrees in Psychology and Special Education at the University of Utah and spent many years as a teacher and case manager working with children and adults with disabilities. She suffers from the rare and disabling mineral metabolic disorder called Periodic Paralysis.

Calvin, the Primary Director of PPNI, earned B.S. degrees in Behavioral Science and Psychology at Westminster College and the University of Utah. He also holds a M.Ed. degree in Special Education and M.S. degree in Information Technology from the University of Utah and Capella University. Calvin worked in a variety of fields including teaching, corrections and case management.

Calvin and Susan have co-authored and co-published four books; *living with Periodic Paralysis: The Mystery Unraveled*, *The Periodic Paralysis Guide and Workbook*: Be The Best You Can Be Naturally, *Sotos Syndrome: A Tribute to Sandy* and *Moments In Time: At Home In The Woods*.

The tree reflects the single "Tree of Life" those of us with Periodic Paralysis share. The earth signifies the elements: potassium, magnesium, sodium, etc. The broken earth signifies the break in those for us. Created by Calvin Hunter.
Periodic Paralysis Network, Inc
Copyright © 2014

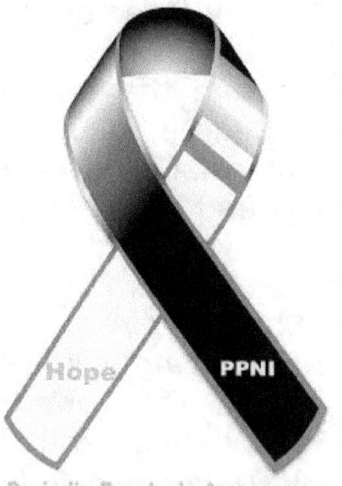

The Awareness Ribbon for Periodic Paralysis is cream and silver. Cream is the color of the Awareness Ribbon for paralysis and silver is the color of potassium. Created by Susan Q. Knittle-Hunter.
Periodic Paralysis Network, Inc
Copyright © 2014

Notes

Notes

www.ingramcontent.com/pod-product-compliance
Lightning Source LLC
Chambersburg PA
CBHW062011280526
45787CB00005B/2062